Nursing & Health Survival Guide

Diabetes

Erica Whettem

Routledge
Taylor & Francis Group

LONDON AND NEW YORK

First published 2012 by Pearson Education Limited

Published 2014 by Routledge
2 Park Square, Milton Park, Abingdon, Oxon OX14 4RN
711 Third Avenue, New York, NY 10017, USA

Routledge is an imprint of the Taylor & Francis Group, an informa business

Copyright © 2012, Taylor & Francis.

ISBN 13: 978-0-273-75801-3 (hbk)

British Library Cataloguing-in-Publication Data
A catalogue record for this book is available from the British Library

Library of Congress Cataloging-in-Publication Data
A catalog record for this book is available from the Library of Congress

Typeset in 8/9.5pt Helvetica by 35

contents

In every setting, in every specialism and at every level, you will encounter growing numbers of people with diabetes throughout your working life as the condition escalates worldwide.

Each contact represents an opportunity to promote good diabetes management, to optimise glycaemic control and to prevent unnecessary complications, but diabetes is well-recognised as a complex and challenging condition.

In a practical easy-to-use quick-reference format, this *Diabetes Survival Guide* provides essential at-a-glance guidance to enable you to deliver proactive day-to-day diabetes care competently and confidently, directly improving health outcomes, experiences and quality of life for people with diabetes.

The book's primary orientation is diabetes in adults, but cross-branch considerations are explored.

Note: Underlining in the text denotes a cross-reference to <u>another section</u> (page number as shown in parenthesis).

Diabetes basics

Diabetes, more properly diabetes mellitus, is a complex chronic metabolic/endocrine disorder characterised by loss of normal <u>blood glucose regulation</u> (p.1) and <u>hyperglycaemia</u> (p.33).

■ BLOOD GLUCOSE REGULATION

Glucose derived from the <u>diet</u> (p.9) is the body's main source of energy. Blood glucose levels are regulated by the pancreas.

Beta cells within the pancreas produce the hormone <u>insulin</u> (p.19). By activating insulin receptors in cell walls, insulin enables the body's tissues to take up circulating glucose for use as energy or for storage as glycogen in the liver/muscles. The beta cells secrete a steady supply of background (basal) insulin, ensuring availability of glucose to tissues at all times, with an extra burst (bolus) of insulin output in response to a glucose load.

Low blood glucose levels, e.g. during fasting periods or <u>exercise</u> (p.16), trigger secretion of another hormone, glucagon, from the alpha cells in the pancreas. Glucagon stimulates the release of glucose from stored glycogen in the liver/muscles back into the bloodstream for use as energy.

Blood glucose levels vary throughout the day and from person to person, with the normal fasting range 3.5–5.9 mmol/L. Blood glucose regulation is governed by negative feedback.

Figure 1 Blood glucose regulation

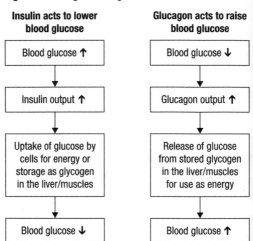

■ TYPES OF DIABETES

In diabetes, factors compromising normal <u>blood glucose regulation</u> (p.1) are:
- insulin deficiency – a problem with insulin production
- insulin resistance – reduced sensitivity to the action of insulin.

The two main types of diabetes are <u>type 1 diabetes</u> (p.3) and <u>type 2 diabetes</u> (p.3). The old terms 'insulin-dependent' and 'non-insulin-dependent' diabetes no longer apply and should not be used. There are no 'mild' forms of diabetes.

Type 1 diabetes

Type 1 diabetes is an autoimmune/idiopathic disorder where the pancreatic beta cells are destroyed and the ability to produce insulin is lost, causing absolute insulin deficiency. This is a life-threatening condition, often with acute presentation (<u>diabetic ketoacidosis [DKA]</u> (p.35)), that requires lifelong <u>insulin</u> (p.19) therapy for survival, alongside a healthy <u>lifestyle</u> (p.8). Type 1 diabetes typically occurs in <u>children and young people</u> (p.47) but can occur in older people.

Around 10–15% of people with diabetes have type 1 diabetes. It is thought to result from a combination of genetic (a first-degree relative with type 1 diabetes increases the risk) and environmental (e.g. viral, chemical) factors. Other autoimmune conditions are more common in people with type 1 diabetes, including coeliac and thyroid disease.

Type 2 diabetes

Type 2 diabetes is a progressive condition characterised by insulin resistance and relative insulin deficiency. Onset is usually more gradual than <u>type 1 diabetes</u> (p.3) and may go undetected for several years, leading to the development of <u>long-term complications</u> (p.44) prior to <u>diagnosis</u> (p.6). <u>Lifestyle</u> (p.8) interventions form the foundation of care, with the addition of <u>medication</u> (p.19), including insulin, as required for <u>glycaemic control</u> (p.30).

The commonest cause of insulin resistance is obesity – 80–90% of people with type 2 diabetes are over<u>weight</u> (p.17) at diagnosis. Insulin production continues but typically declines over time. The majority of people with diabetes have type 2 (85–90%). It is more common in people of South Asian, African and Afro-Caribbean origin, and in people with a family history of the disease. Previously regarded as mature-onset, with escalating obesity levels type 2 diabetes is now presenting in younger people, including growing numbers of children. It is often preceded by a state of impaired glucose regulation (p.6).

Other types of diabetes

Diabetes can be *secondary* to pancreatic impairment due to surgery (pancreatectomy) and conditions such as cystic fibrosis, pancreatitis and haemochromatosis.

Gestational diabetes is a first diagnosis of diabetes in pregnancy (p.50). It usually resolves post-delivery but women who experience gestational diabetes are at risk of developing type 2 diabetes (p.3) in later life.

Monogenic diabetes is caused by a mutation in a single gene. Affecting just 1–2% of diabetes cases, the main forms of monogenic diabetes are:

- Maturity-Onset Diabetes of the Young (MODY) – inherited diabetes usually diagnosed between the ages of 5 and 30
- Neonatal diabetes – transient or permanent diabetes diagnosed before the age of 6 months (new mutation).

■ SYMPTOMS OF DIABETES

The symptoms of diabetes are the symptoms of hyperglycaemia (p.33). They are reversible and will resolve once normal blood glucose levels are restored. Experience of hyperglycaemic symptoms can be very individual.

SYMPTOM	REASON
Polyuria, especially nocturia	When blood glucose levels exceed the renal threshold for reabsorption (usually around 10 mmol/L), the result is glycosuria with osmotic diuresis, occasionally leading to bedwetting in children and incontinence in older people
Polydipsia	Response to dehydration from osmotic diuresis
Fatigue	Reduced glucose uptake by cells 'starves' the body of energy; fatigue is not helped by nocturia
Blurred vision	Increased levels of glucose and its metabolites within the lens lead to lens swelling and visual distortion
Recurrent infections/poor healing	Hyperglycaemia impairs the action of neutrophils, muting the body's immune response to infection, while infective organisms can thrive on a prolific energy source
Pins and needles	Hyperglycaemia can cause peripheral nerve irritation
Weight loss	Where insulin deficiency prevents normal glucose uptake, the body breaks down fat reserves in a bid to obtain energy, producing ketones (p.33)
No symptoms	It is not clear why some people have no awareness of hyperglycaemia

Be alert to symptoms of hyperglycaemia and ensure they are followed up promptly, whether people are known to have diabetes or not.

■ DIAGNOSIS

In the UK, diagnostic criteria follow World Health Organization guidelines (WHO 2006, 2011).

Diabetes

Where symptoms of diabetes (p.4) are present, a diagnosis may be made on the basis of one of the following:

- Random venous plasma glucose of ≥11.1 mmol/L
- Fasting venous plasma glucose of ≥7.0 mmol/L
- Venous plasma glucose of ≥11.1 mmol/L 2 hours after a 75g oral glucose tolerance test (p.7)
- HbA$_{1c}$ (p.30) of ≥48 mmol/mol (6.5%) (conditions apply).

In the absence of symptoms, repeat testing on a different day is required to confirm diagnosis.

Impaired glucose regulation

People who have higher than normal blood glucose levels but do not yet meet the criteria for a diagnosis of diabetes have impaired glucose regulation and are at increased risk of developing type 2 diabetes (p.3).

- *Impaired fasting glucose* is defined as a fasting venous plasma glucose of 6.1–6.9 mmol/L and (if measured) 2-hour post-glucose load of <7.8 mmol/L
- *Impaired glucose tolerance* is defined as a fasting blood glucose of <7.0 mmol/L but 2-hour level of 7.8–11.0 mmol/L (oral glucose tolerance test (p.7)).

Evidence suggests intensive underlined_lifestyle (p.8) interventions can significantly delay the onset of diabetes in people with impaired glucose regulation.

Oral glucose tolerance test

An oral glucose tolerance test (OGTT) measures fasting venous plasma glucose prior to a 75g oral glucose load, then measures venous plasma glucose again 2 hours later. The patient should eat/exercise normally in the days preceding the test, drink water only for 8–12 hours immediately before the test and sit quietly/refrain from smoking during the test. An OGTT is the only means of diagnosing impaired glucose tolerance.

■ COMPLICATIONS

Diabetes not only carries the risk of acute short-term complications, such as diabetic ketoacidosis (DKA) (p.35), hyperosmolar hyperglycaemic state (HHS) (p.36) and hypoglycaemia (p.38), it is also associated with a range of disabling and life-threatening long-term complications (p.44).

Diabetes management

Aimed at optimising glycaemic control (p.30) and preventing long-term complications (p.44), front-line diabetes care is provided by GP surgeries working in conjunction with specialist teams of diabetes consultants, nurses, dietitians, podiatrists and psychologists spanning primary and secondary care, and including dedicated multidisciplinary paediatric teams. Familiarise yourself with the referral pathways/contact details relevant to your area and consider spending time with specialist colleagues.

■ SELF-MANAGEMENT

Good diabetes management involves partnership between healthcare providers and individuals with diabetes actively managing their condition themselves on a day-to-day basis, a role which may extend to family, friends and carers/ support workers in the case of children and young people (p.47), older people (p.49) and people with learning disabilities or mental health problems.

There are structured education programmes to help people with diabetes develop the knowledge, skills and confidence they need to self-manage diabetes effectively but everyone in healthcare has a role to play by providing support, recognising problems, making appropriate referrals and offering accurate up-to-date information/advice on:

- lifestyle (p.8)
- medication (p.19)
- glycaemic control (p.30)
- long-term complications (p.44)
- life with diabetes (p.47).

For guidance on goal-setting and behaviour change, see the *Student Nurse Health Promotion Survival Guide* (Upton 2010).

■ LIFESTYLE

Healthy living is the foundation of care in all types of diabetes (p.2). Modification of lifestyle in people at high risk of developing type 2 diabetes (p.3) can help prevent its onset and should be encouraged.

Diet

There is no such thing as a diabetic diet – healthy eating advice for people with diabetes is the same as for people without.

- Balanced diet with regular meals including starchy <u>carbohydrates</u> (p.9)
- Low sugar
- At least 5 portions of fruit/vegetables a day
- High in <u>fibre</u> (p.12)
- Low in <u>fat</u> (p.12), especially saturates
- Two portions of oily fish a week
- Low in <u>salt</u> (p.14)
- Moderate <u>alcohol</u> (p.14) consumption.

Diabetic products are not recommended – they are expensive, often quite high in <u>fat</u> (p.12) and may be sweetened with sorbitol, which can cause diarrhoea.

Everyone newly diagnosed with diabetes should have access to a dietitian with follow-up dietetic input as required.

Carbohydrates

Figure 2 The action of carbohydrates

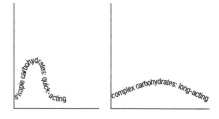

Carbohydrates are the only food group that will break down to glucose in digestion. Because of their molecular structure, simple carbohydrates (sugars) require very little digestion and are therefore absorbed into the bloodstream very quickly, causing a sharp rise in blood glucose. These quick-acting carbohydrates are important for treating hypoglycaemia (p.38) but are otherwise best kept to a minimum.

FOR ...	SUBSTITUTE ...
Sugar	Sweetener
Jam/marmalade	Reduced-sugar versions
Sweets	Sugar-free sweets
Fizzy drinks/squash	Diet/no added sugar

Conversely, complex or starchy carbohydrates take longer for the body to digest and are therefore absorbed more gradually, giving a flatter longer-lasting blood glucose profile, providing sustained energy without causing spikes. Most staple foods come into this category.

Higher fibre (p.12) varieties of long-acting carbohydrates are especially good for slowing the absorption of glucose, though even these, eaten in sufficient quantity, will cause a rise in blood glucose.

STARCHY CARBOHYDRATES	BEST CHOICE – HIGH FIBRE
Potatoes	New, boiled in their skins
Pasta	All good
Rice	Wholegrain, basmati
Bread	Granary
Pulses	All good
Cereals	Oats, wholegrain
Flour	Wholegrain

All high-sugar products, such as chocolate, cakes, biscuits and puddings, will cause a rise in blood glucose levels and are often also high in fat (p.12) and therefore high in calories. If weight (p.17) is not an issue, a couple of squares of chocolate after a meal (which will delay their absorption) and plainer/reduced-sugar varieties of cakes, biscuits and puddings are acceptable in moderation.

Fruit contains its own natural sugar, fructose, which may raise blood glucose levels if consumed in large quantities, but it is a healthy snack high in fibre (p.12) and rich in cardioprotective antioxidants. All fruit is acceptable, including bananas and grapes. The key is to keep intake to a portion at a time (roughly what you can hold in your hand) and spread consumption through the day. A good mix of fruit is also important.

- Take care with fruit juice as it contains the concentrated sugar of several pieces of fruit with none of the fibre of the whole fruit – stick to a single small glass a day with a meal
- Take care with dried fruit, as only moisture not sugar is lost in the drying process
- Avoid tinned fruit in syrup.

Milk and milk-products such as yoghurts also contain their own natural sugar, lactose, which again can contribute to a rise in blood glucose levels in sufficient quantities. However, milk and no-added-sugar dairy products spread throughout the day are an important source of calcium.

By ranking carbohydrates according to their effect on blood glucose levels, the glycaemic index (GI) can be a useful guide but it does not take account of the overall amount consumed (glycaemic load), the cooking methods, the impact of any other foodstuffs consumed at the same time or variations in individual response.

Fibre

A high-fibre diet is important for bowel function and for cardiovascular health. Fibre slows down the absorption of glucose from the diet, and foods high in soluble fibre, such as pulses, oats, fruit and vegetables, can help lower cholesterol. A high-fibre diet can also help control weight (p.17) through satiety.

Fat

The two main types of dietary fat are saturates and unsaturates. Saturated fat is mainly animal-derived and typically hard at room temperature (e.g. cheese, butter, fat on meat, cream, lard, dripping). Unsaturated fat, generally found in plant foods, including nuts and seeds, divides into monounsaturates (e.g. olive oil/spread, rapeseed oil – often marketed as vegetable oil) and polyunsaturates (e.g. sunflower oil/spread, groundnut oil, corn oil, soya oil, sesame oil).

Monounsaturated fat is considered the best choice because it can lower 'bad' low-density lipoprotein (LDL) cholesterol while raising 'good' high-density lipoprotein (HDL) cholesterol. Polyunsaturated fat will also lower cholesterol but tends to lower both LDL and HDL cholesterol while saturated fat is associated with raised LDL levels, a major risk factor for cardiovascular disease (long-term complications (p.44)).

Because of its role in the development of atherosclerosis, a reduction in saturated fat is particularly recommended but all fat is high in calories – approximately 9 kcal/g compared with 4 kcal/g for carbohydrate and protein – so for weight (p.17) control a reduction of total fat intake is important.

- Be careful with ready meals and snacks high in fat
- Choose leaner meats and remove visible fat including bacon rind/chicken skin
- Use less fat in cooking – grill or bake and drain fat off
- Use lower fat alternatives such as reduced-fat cheese and skimmed/semi-skimmed milk.

Most of the cholesterol in the body is produced by the liver, not obtained from cholesterol-containing foods such as eggs, shellfish and offal. These may therefore be eaten in moderation and do not need to be avoided.

Oily fish, e.g. salmon, herring, sardines/pilchards, mackerel, trout, crab and tuna, are rich in omega-3 polyunsaturated fatty acids, which have been shown to be beneficial for the heart, joints and brain. For people with diabetes, two portions a week of oily fish are recommended, including tinned varieties for all except tuna, which loses the omega-3 oils in the canning process.

Plant stanols and sterols have also been shown to lower cholesterol and ranges of enriched dairy products are available. They can be expensive, however, and need to be consumed in the specified quantities. There is no benefit if cholesterol levels are not raised.

Salt

Dietary salt intake has been linked to hypertension, heart disease and stroke. The recommended daily limit of 6g, approximately a teaspoon, is commonly exceeded. Salt is found in all foods and can be particularly high in processed foods, ready meals and take-aways.

Cutting down on salt used in cooking and not adding at the table can help reduce overall intake. Alternatives such as herbs, spices, lemon juice, garlic and pepper can be used for flavouring. Salt substitutes are best avoided – they are potassium-based rather than sodium-based and are therefore contraindicated with cardiac/renal problems. Also, they do not allow the taste buds to adjust to less salt in the diet.

Alcohol

The recommended guidelines for people with diabetes are the same as for those without – 2–3 units a day for women and 3–4 units a day for men, with some alcohol-free days in the week.

One unit is approximately:

- half a pint of lager, beer, cider
- two-thirds of a small glass (125ml) of wine
- a pub measure (25ml) of spirit.

Because the alcoholic strength of many beers and wines has increased since units were first calculated, and so has the size of wine glasses, drinks often contain more units than meets the eye.

It is never a good idea to drink on an empty stomach. In people on <u>insulin</u> (p.19)/sulphonylurea <u>tablets</u> (p.26), intake in excess of recommended guidelines can cause delayed <u>hypoglycaemia</u> (p.38) up to 16 hours later and the consumption of food with/after alcohol should be encouraged.

Some alcoholic drinks contain carbohydrate (beer, cider, alcopops, liqueurs), which may cause an initial rise in blood glucose, but low-carbohydrate varieties tend to contain more alcohol so are not a better choice. Recommend sugar free mixers.

Apart from the general health problems associated with excess consumption, alcohol also contains high levels of 'empty calories' (7kcal/g) and can contribute to <u>weight</u> (p.17) problems.

Food labels

The simplest way to evaluate a product is to look at the Ingredients list, which presents items in descending order of quantity. A more accurate way is to look at the ingredients per 100g column. This provides content information as a percentage, which can then be used in conjunction with the amount of the product that will be consumed to determine whether or not it is a healthy choice.

	LOW (PER 100g)	HIGH (PER 100g)
Sugars	≤5g	>15g
Fat	≤3g	>20g
Saturates	≤1.5g	>5g
Salt	≤0.3g	>1.5g
Fibre	–	≥6g

Labels can be misleading:
- The amount of sugar per 100g does not differentiate between added sugar and natural sugar – if the product is high in added sugar, sugar will appear at the beginning of the ingredients list
- 'Reduced fat' simply means 25% less than the original product and 'low-fat' products can often be high in sugar
- Salt is sodium chloride but manufacturers sometimes list its equivalent as sodium, which is 2.5 times lower than sodium chloride.

Exercise
Exercise can help 'burn off' blood glucose by using it as energy. Regular <u>physical activity</u> (p.50) can increase insulin sensitivity and improve <u>glycaemic control</u> (p.30). It can also have a

beneficial effect on blood pressure and cholesterol, <u>weight</u> (p.17) and mood. Current recommendations for adults are for at least 30 minutes of moderate activity 5 days a week, not necessarily in a single stretch, with at least an hour a day for children.

Moderate activity is defined as causing slight breathlessness and covers housework, shopping, gardening and leisure pursuits such as dancing as well as all forms of sport.

Encourage people to take simple steps such as getting off the bus a stop earlier and walking, using the stairs instead of the lift and parking further from the supermarket entrance. For people with limited mobility, simple chair-based exercises can be helpful. For more structured exercise programmes, choosing an enjoyable activity will help maintain motivation. It is a good idea for anyone with complex health problems to consult their doctor before commencing.

Weight

Excess weight, particularly with central obesity, is associated with many serious health problems, including heart disease and stroke (<u>long-term complications</u> (p.44)), osteoarthritis and some cancers. It is a major factor in the development of <u>type 2 diabetes</u> (p.3), causing insulin resistance and eventually insulin deficiency.

Figure 3 Central obesity is associated with insulin resistance

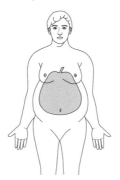

A healthy weight is currently defined as a body mass index (BMI) of 18.5–24.9kg/m² with a waist circumference of <94cm for a man (<90cm for South Asian men) and <80cm for a woman. A healthy <u>diet</u> (p.9), portion control and regular <u>exercise</u> (p.16) all play a role in weight management.

Growing numbers of people of all ages are now categorised as obese (BMI ≥ 30kg/m²). Recommend steady weight loss over time – a target of 0.5–1kg a week, equivalent to a 600 kcal/day deficit, will generally be easier to maintain. Losing 5–10% of body weight can significantly improve <u>glycaemic control</u> (p.30) and health outcomes, but even lesser amounts can be beneficial.

Smoking

Smoking is associated with many health problems in its own right. With diabetes, it significantly increases the risk of developing cardiovascular disease (long-term complications (p.44)). Reinforce the importance of quitting for current and future health and provide appropriate information on cessation support.

■ MEDICATION

The aim of diabetes medication is to control hyperglycaemia (p.33) and prevent long-term complications (p.44). New generations of diabetes medications continue to become available. For detailed prescribing information, consult the *British National Formulary* (www.bnf.org.uk).

Insulin

Everyone with type 1 diabetes (p.3) is dependent on insulin and some people with type 2 diabetes (p.3) also require insulin (this does not mean they have developed type 1 diabetes). There are several different types of insulin/regimen (p.20), depending on individual needs and lifestyles, and insulin doses may vary enormously from person to person. It is essential that the correct insulin is received at the correct dose, at the correct time and in the correct way.

As a general rule insulin should never be omitted, although a reduced dose may sometimes be appropriate (hypoglycaemia (p.38), physical activity (p.50)). Omitting insulin in type 1 diabetes (p.3) can precipitate life-threatening diabetic ketoacidosis (DKA) (p.35).

Types of insulin/regimen

The first insulin available for human use was animal-derived and porcine/bovine insulins are still available today. Human insulins were then developed and have become the mainstay of treatment with the more recent arrival of analogues using recombinant DNA technology to modify their absorption properties.

There are many ways of describing different insulins but, broadly speaking, they fall into three main categories:

1. Background insulin
2. Mealtime insulin
3. Mixed insulin.

Background insulin, also known as *basal* insulin, provides background cover in once- or twice-daily injections, usually in conjunction with mealtime insulin in a basal–bolus regimen or with other therapies (p.26) in type 2 diabetes (p.3). Long-acting analogues are clear in appearance and have a longer, steadier, more stable release (onset 1–2 hours, duration up to 24 hours) than the intermediate human insulins, which are cloudy, require resuspension through thorough gentle mixing before administration, take more time to become fully active and rise to a gentle peak before falling away (onset 45–60 minutes, main action 4–12 hours, duration up to 24 hours). Because of its action profile, people on intermediate human insulin may need a midmeal/bedtime snack (plain biscuits, toast, cereal) to prevent hypoglycaemia (p.38).

NAME	TYPE	TIMING
Humulin® I	Intermediate human	Usually bedtime/evening and/or morning
Insulatard®	Intermediate human	Usually bedtime/evening and/or morning
Insuman® Basal	Intermediate human	Usually bedtime/evening and/or morning
Lantus®	Long-acting analogue	Once daily (within an hour of the same time)
Levemir®	Long-acting analogue	Once or twice daily (within an hour of the same time[s])

Mealtime insulin, also known as *prandial* or *bolus* insulin, covers the carbohydrates (p.9) in meals, usually in three injections a day but more/less often if eating patterns are variable. There are rapid-acting analogues and short-acting human insulins, both of which are clear in appearance. They are usually combined with once- or twice-daily background insulin in a basal bolus regimen. Rapid-acting analogues have a quicker/shorter profile of action (onset 10–15 minutes, main action 2–3 hours, duration up to 5 hours) than the short-acting human insulins (onset 30–60 minutes, main action up to 6 hours, duration up to 8 hours) and are therefore injected closer to meals.

NAME	TYPE	TIMING
Actrapid®	Short-acting human	30 mins before eating
Apidra®	Rapid-acting analogue	0–15 minutes before, during or just after eating
Humalog®	Rapid-acting analogue	Immediately before, during or just after eating
Humulin® S	Short-acting human	20–45 minutes before eating
Insuman® Rapid	Short-acting human	15–20 minutes before eating
NovoRapid®	Rapid-acting analogue	Immediately before, during or just after eating

Mixed insulin, also known as *premixed* or *biphasic* insulin, provides a fixed proportion of background and mealtime insulin combined, usually in twice-daily injections before breakfast and evening meal. Mixed insulins are cloudy and require resuspension through thorough gentle mixing before administration. Because of their quicker onset, mixes based on analogue insulins are injected closer to meals. A midmeal/bedtime snack to prevent hypoglycaemia (p.38) (plain biscuits, toast, cereal) is more likely to be required with human insulin mixes because of their action profile.

NAME	TYPE	TIMING
Humalog® Mix 25	Analogue mix (25% rapid-acting)	Immediately before, during or just after eating
Humalog® Mix 50	Analogue mix (50% rapid-acting)	Immediately before, during or just after eating
Humulin® M3	Human mix (30% short-acting)	20–45 minutes before eating
Insuman® Comb 15	Human mix (15% short-acting)	30–45 minutes before eating
Insuman® Comb 25	Human mix (25% short-acting)	30–45 minutes before eating
Insuman® Comb 50	Human mix (50% short-acting)	20–30 minutes before eating
NovoMix® 30	Analogue mix (30% rapid-acting)	Immediately before, during or just after eating

Basal–bolus regimens using multiple daily injections (MDI) aim to replicate the physiology of normal blood glucose regulation (p.1) as closely as possible and offer the greatest flexibility. Mixed insulin aims to provide similar cover with fewer daily injections but works best in people with regular routines.

People with type 1 diabetes (p.3) on a basal–bolus regimen, or their parents in the case of children, often learn to 'carbohydrate count' so they can accurately adjust insulin doses around their planned intake of carbohydrates (p.9) and exercise (p.16)/physical activity (p.50). They also learn how to calculate correction doses for hyperglycaemia (p.33) using their mealtime insulin.

Administration

Insulin injections should normally be made at a 90° angle into subcutaneous tissue by means of an insulin syringe or pen device. Because of the risk of needlestick injury, pens are only recommended for self-injection, not for injections to a third party.

Insulin pens are specific to particular insulin(s). Some are disposable and some are refillable with cartridges. Needles come in a variety of lengths but research now suggests that shorter needles (4–6mm) are suitable for most people.

- Use a new needle for each injection to avoid discomfort and reduce the risk of tissue microtrauma at <u>injection sites</u> (p.25)
- Before injecting, hold the pen vertically with the needle uppermost and 'prime' the pen by means of a 2-unit 'airshot' (repeat until drops are visible at the end of the needle)
- For less fleshy sites/longer needles, 'pinch up' to ensure delivery into subcutaneous tissue rather than muscle, which can accelerate the drug's release and is more painful
- Never inject through clothing – this is unhygienic and it is impossible to see that the injection has been given properly
- Following injection, leave the pen *in situ* for 6–10 seconds before withdrawal to ensure the full dose is received and absorbed
- Never leave a needle on the pen between injections as this allows insulin to leak out of the cartridge (potentially altering its concentration) and air to be drawn in (potentially altering its mode of action)
- Always dispose of sharps safely

Increasing numbers of people, including children, are now using continuous subcutaneous insulin infusion (CSII) pumps. Any queries about these should be directed to the diabetes team.

Injection sites

Figure 4 Subcutaneous injection sites

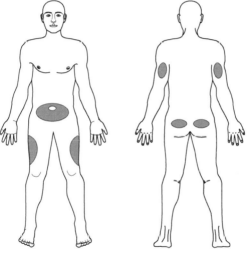

It is very important to rotate injection sites, moving from one to another and within the same site. Repeated use of the same site can lead to the development of fatty lumps – lipohypertrophy or 'lipos' for short – in subcutaneous tissue. Reusing needles can also contribute to lipos, which not only look unsightly but can affect the absorption of insulin, causing erratic blood glucose (p.42) levels. They are not always visible but can be felt by running a finger across the site area.

The abdomen offers the quickest, most predictable absorption. Unless fleshy, arms are no longer recommended for self-injection because of the risk of injecting into muscle, and thighs are best avoided if physical activity is planned as the increased blood flow can accelerate insulin absorption.

Storage

Once open, all insulin is safe to use for one month. Current insulin should be kept at room temperature, with unopened supplies stored in the fridge (2–8°C).

Side effects

Insulin can cause hypoglycaemia (p.38) and weight (p.17) gain.

Other therapies

Type 2 diabetes (p.3) may be controlled through diet (p.9) and exercise (p.16) alone or in conjunction with diabetes medication. The progressive nature of type 2 diabetes usually requires therapy intensification over time, including insulin (p.19) initiation in some people.

Tablets

Different classes of diabetes tablets work in different ways. It is important that the correct tablets are received at the correct dose at the correct time.

The usual first-/second-line tablets in type 2 diabetes are metformin and/or a sulphonylurea (usually gliclazide in the UK) as mono or dual therapy. Both have a long history of common use in people with type 2 diabetes. Meglitinides are a rarely used alternative to sulphonylureas.

		(GLICLAZIDE, GLIMEPIRIDE, GLIPIZIDE, TOLBUTAMIDE)	(REPAGLINIDE, NATEGLINIDE)
Timing	With or after meals	With meals	Just before main meals
Action	Reduces insulin resistance, increases peripheral glucose uptake, reduces glucose absorption and reduces inappropriate hepatic glucose output	Augments insulin secretion	Augments insulin secretion
Side effects	Gastrointestinal (GI) disturbances	Hypoglycaemia (p.38), weight (p.17) gain	Hypoglycaemia (p.3E), weight (p.17) gain
Notes	Can be used with all other diabetes tablets as well as with glucagon-like peptide-1 (GLP-1) analogues (p.28) and insulin (p.19). Cardioprotective, weight (p.17) neutral, does not usually cause hypoglycaemia (p.38). Can cause lactic acidosis, particularly in people with renal impairment, and should be reviewed if glomerular filtration rate is <45 ml/min/1.73m². Usually stopped for 48 hours or tests involving radio-opaque contrast media. The once-daily slow-release version (Glucophage® SR) may help GI side effects. Sometimes used in people with type 1 diabetes (p.3) who have a BMI >25 kg/m² (weight (p.17).	May be used with metformin and insulin (p.19) or DPP-4 inhibitors/pioglitazone. There is a once-daily modified-release version of gliclazide (Diamicron® MR).	The quicker shorter action profile compared with sulphonylureas targets post-prandial hyperglycaemia (p.33) with less risk of hypoglycaemia (p.3E).

The newer agents, pioglitazone and the dipeptidyl peptidase-4 (DPP-4) inhibitors (also known as gliptins), are typically second-/third-line treatments.

	PIOGLITAZONE	DPP-4 INHIBITORS (LINAGLIPTIN, SAXAGLIPTIN, SITAGLIPTIN, VILDAGLIPTIN)
Timing	With or without food	With or without food
Action	Reduces insulin resistance, increases peripheral glucose uptake	Blocks the action of the DPP-4 enzyme, increasing insulin secretion in response to ingested glucose and reducing glucagon secretion
Side effects	<u>Weight</u> (p.17) gain, fluid retention, GI disturbances	GI disturbances, peripheral oedema
Notes	Can be used with metformin (Competact®) and/ or a sulphonylurea; use with <u>insulin</u> (p.19) subject to cardiac status	See *British National Formulary* for licensed use of individual drugs (www.bnf.org.uk)

Glucagon-like peptide-1 (GLP-1) analogues

Given by subcutaneous injection, GLP-1 analogues are for obese individuals (primarily BMI >35 kg/m^2) with type 2 diabetes whose <u>glycaemic control</u> (p.30) is inadequate on maximum diabetes <u>tablets</u> (p.26). Also known as incretin mimetics, they increase insulin secretion in response to ingested glucose, inhibit glucagon secretion, reduce appetite and delay gastric emptying, reducing blood glucose and promoting weight loss. Their main side effect is nausea/vomiting, which usually resolves with time. They may be used with metformin and/or a sulphonylurea/pioglitazone (tablets (p.26)).

The first GLP-1 analogues on the market were:

Exenatide	Byetta®	Prefilled pen	Taken twice a day within 1 hour before the two main meals of the day (at least 6 hours apart)
	Bydureon®	Prefilled syringe with powder for suspension	Prolonged release taken once a week at any time of day with or without food
Liraglutide	Victoza®	Prefilled pen	Taken once a day at any time of day with or without food

■ ANNUAL REVIEW

Regular annual review is a core element of diabetes management. Its purpose is to:

- monitor clinical parameters
- assess lifestyle (p.8) and provide self-management (p.8) support
- optimise diabetes medication (p.19)/glycaemic control (p.30)

- screen for <u>long-term complications</u> (p.44)
- set goals and agree an individualised care plan.

Interim reviews should be conducted as often as is required to address specific aspects of diabetes care as they occur. Encourage people to attend these important reviews.

Glycaemic control

Optimising glycaemic control to prevent <u>hyperglycaemia</u> (p.33), <u>hypoglycaemia</u> (p.38) and <u>long-term complications</u> (p.44) is an essential ongoing process and a key aim of <u>diabetes management</u> (p.7), involving careful <u>monitoring</u> (p.30) and <u>medication</u> (p.19) adjustment in response to a range of variables.

■ MONITORING

Monitoring methods, frequency and targets should be appropriate to the individual and adjusted in response to changing circumstances.

HbA$_{1c}$

Long-term glycaemic control is monitored by HbA$_{1c}$, a venous blood test that measures the amount of glucose bound to the haemoglobin in red blood cells, providing an overview of the preceding 2–3 months (the lifespan of a red blood cell). HbA$_{1c}$ is measured in mmol/mol (it was previously measured as a percentage) and is normally around 31 mmol/mol (5%). The lower the HbA$_{1c}$, the lower the risk of <u>long-term complications</u> (p.44) but the higher the risk of <u>hypoglycaemia</u> (p.38).

Target

The target for HbA$_{1c}$ is usually between 48 and 58 mmol/mol (6.5–7.5%) but tight control is not appropriate for everyone with diabetes or in all circumstances and people should have individualised HbA_{1c} targets that take personal factors into account (annual review (p.29)).

Frequency

HbA_{1c} should be measured at least 6-monthly, more frequently at periods of instability or medication (p.19) change.

Capillary blood glucose (CBG)

Many people with diabetes self-monitor their day-to-day glycaemic control by CBG (finger prick) testing using a glucometer, a function often taken over by staff in a hospital or care setting, by carers in the community and by parents of children with diabetes. A CBG test measures (in mmol/L) the amount of glucose in the bloodstream at the time of the test. Some glucometers can also measure blood ketones (p.33). Glucometers should be calibrated according to manufacturers' instructions/local protocols.

Target

The general pre-meal CBG target for people with diabetes is 4–7 mmol/L (4–8 mmol/L for children with type 1 diabetes). Like HbA_{1c} (p.30), however, CBG targets should be appropriate to individuals and their circumstances.

Frequency

People with type 2 diabetes (p.3) that is well controlled without medication (p.19) do not routinely need to test their blood glucose levels (HbA_{1c} (p.30)), although for those newly diagnosed it is a useful tool for exploring the effects of diet (p.9) and exercise (p.16). Conversely, people on a basal–bolus insulin (p.19) regimen need to test their blood glucose levels regularly throughout the day, whether they are well controlled or not.

Generally the more complex someone's diabetes medication (p.19) and the poorer their glycaemic control, the more frequently they need to test, usually four times a day before meals and before bed but more frequently at other times (sick-day rules (p.37), hypoglycaemia (p.38), physical activity (p.50)). The diabetes team can advise on this.

Because self-monitoring CBG represents a significant NHS overhead, encourage people to test responsibly and act appropriately on their results, seeking advice promptly if unsure of what action to take themselves.

- Always wash hands with soap and water (not alcohol or wipes) and dry thoroughly before testing
- Avoid the thumb and index finger to preserve sensitivity
- Test along the side of the fingerpad – this can be less painful and preserves sensitivity in the fingertip
- Set the finger-pricker to deliver only the amount of blood required for the test strip
- Squeezing the finger too hard to get blood out can give a false reading – often waiting a few seconds after pricking and gently 'milking' the finger by stroking down its length will encourage the blood to flow
- Warming the hand before testing and holding the arm with the hand down for a few minutes can also improve blood flow
- Change the lancet for each test and always dispose of sharps safely
- Write readings in a record diary – this makes it easier to interpret the blood glucose profile across the day

Urinalysis

Non-invasive and convenient, dipstick urinalysis can detect rises in both blood glucose and ketones (p.33).

Glycosuria is indicative of an above normal blood glucose level, usually >10 mmol/L, and should not be ignored, although dipstick urinalysis cannot accurately reflect the timing/degree of the rise or detect hypoglycaemia (p.38), unlike capillary blood glucose (CBG) (p.31) testing. Ketonuria with glycosuria should always be followed up because of the risk of diabetic ketoacidosis (DKA) (p.35).

Ketones

Ketones are weak organic acids produced when the body metabolises fat for energy. If fat breakdown is triggered by insulin deficiency preventing glucose uptake, ketones can build up in the blood and lead to diabetic ketoacidosis (DKA) (p.35). People with significant hyperglycaemia (p.33), especially people not known to have diabetes and people with known type 1 diabetes (p.3), should be monitored for ketones and their detection on urinalysis (p.33) (++) or in the blood (>1.6 mmol/L) should be followed up promptly. Ketones sometimes cause an acetone or 'pear drop' smell on the breath.

■ HYPERGLYCAEMIA

Hyperglycaemia should not be ignored. Apart from causing unpleasant symptoms of diabetes (p.4), untreated hyperglycaemia can lead to the medical emergencies of diabetic ketoacidosis (DKA) (p.35) and hyperosmolar hyperglycaemic state (HHS) (p.36) as well as long-term complications (p.44).

Causes of hyperglycaemia

Obvious causes of hyperglycaemia include:

- undiagnosed diabetes
- inadequate diabetes <u>medication</u> (p.19) prescribed
- omission or under-administration (wrong dose) of diabetes medication
- inadequate or delayed diabetes <u>medication</u> (p.19) in relation to <u>carbohydrates</u> (p.9)
- reduced <u>exercise</u> (p.16)/<u>physical activity</u> (p.50).

Other causes include:

- *Steroids* – prescribed for their anti-inflammatory effect, steroids (e.g. prednisolone, dexamethasone) commonly raise blood glucose levels by causing insulin resistance (steroid inhalers/injections should not have this effect)
- *Stress hormones* – stress hormones released in response to illness, infection, surgery and stress/anxiety can raise blood glucose levels, increasing insulin requirements even in people with poor appetite/reduced food intake/vomiting (<u>sick-day rules</u> (p.37))
- <u>*Hypoglycaemia*</u> (p.38) – the combination of the body's release of glucose stores in response to hypoglycaemia and (over)treatment of hypoglycaemia can result in 'rebound' hyperglycaemia
- <u>*Weight*</u> (p.17) *gain* – especially with central obesity because of its association with insulin resistance.

It is important to identify and address the cause(s) of hyperglycaemia. Even temporary patterns of elevation may require <u>medication</u> (p.19) adjustment and <u>self-management</u> (p.8) support. Consider referral to the specialist team.

Diabetic ketoacidosis (DKA)

DKA is characterised by hyperglycaemia, a lack of insulin, fluid/electrolyte disturbance and a build-up in the blood of ketones (p.33). It may be precipitated by an infection or illness and/or by omission of insulin (p.19) injections, and is a life-threatening emergency.

DKA mainly affects people with type 1 diabetes (p.3) but can sometimes affect people with type 2 diabetes (p.3). In people not known to have diabetes, it may be the presenting condition that leads to a diagnosis (p.6). The presence of ketones and glucose on urinalysis (p.33) should always be followed up as a matter of urgency.

Signs and symptoms of DKA (i.e. of progressive hyperglycaemia and acidosis combined) include:

- steadily rising blood glucose levels (≥ 14 mmol/L usually over 24–48 hours)
- polyuria/dehydration
- polydipsia
- tiredness/weakness
- muscle cramps
- abdominal pain
- laboured breathing/breathlessness
- drowsiness/confusion
- nausea/vomiting
- tachycardia/hypotension
- ketones in blood (≥ 3 mmol/L) or urine (+ + +)
- venous bicarbonate <15 mmol/L and/or pH <7.3.

Management involves the treatment of any underlying infection/condition and a combination of insulin and fluid/electrolyte replacement, which usually takes 1–2 days.

Follow-up education with the specialist team is essential to prevent further episodes.

Hyperosmolar hyperglycaemic state (HHS)

HHS predominantly affects older people with type 2 diabetes (p.3), their residual pancreatic function/circulating insulin preventing the development of diabetic ketoacidosis (DKA) (p.35). The onset of HHS is more gradual than DKA but blood glucose levels tend to rise much higher, up to 80 mmol/L. As with DKA, there is often a precipitating illness or infection but HHS may also be the result of undiagnosed diabetes.

HHS is characterised by hyperglycaemia and hyperosmolarity, leading to profound dehydration, fluid/electrolyte disturbance and neurological deficits.

Signs and symptoms include:

- rising blood glucose levels ($\geq$30 mmol/L, usually over days/weeks)
- polyuria/dehydration
- polydipsia/parched mouth
- weight loss
- weakness/shortness of breath on exertion
- confusion
- seizures
- drowsiness/coma
- tachycardia/hypotension.

Like DKA, management combines fluid replacement therapy, insulin and electrolyte restoration with treatment of any underlying infection/condition and follow-up education to prevent further episodes. The mortality rate from HHS is higher than from DKA because of the older age group and frequent presence of complicating co-morbidities.

Sick-day rules

As people with diabetes are unable to compensate for rises in blood glucose levels resulting from illness and infection (causes of hyperglycaemia (p.34)), it is essential that they follow sick-day rules to optimise their glycaemic control and prevent hyperglycaemic emergencies when poorly.

- Never omit diabetes medication (p.19) – blood glucose levels will typically rise during illness, even when food intake is reduced, and diabetes medication may need to be increased
- Test capillary blood glucose (CBG) (p.31) levels frequently – 2–4-hourly if necessary – and adjust medication accordingly
- With type 1 diabetes (p.3) test for ketones (p.33) if blood glucose levels are ≥14 mmol/L – extra insulin (p.19) may be required (this can also happen in type 2 diabetes (p.3))
- Aim to drink 2–3 litres of sugar-free fluid a day
- If appetite is reduced, try replacing solid food with soup, cereals, milk, ice cream, jelly or yoghurt
- If blood glucose levels are dipping and eating is a problem, sip glucose-containing drinks (Lucozade®, fizzy drinks, fruit juices) or suck boiled sweets or glucose tablets in place of usual carbohydrates (p.9)
- Rest to allow time for the body to recover
- Ensure any over-the-counter remedies are sugar-free
- For persistent vomiting/diarrhoea and hyperglycaemia with ketones (p.33), seek medical advice without delay

■ HYPOGLYCAEMIA

A common and feared side effect of insulin (p.19) therapy and sulphonylurea tablets (p.26), hypoglycaemia can become a medical emergency and should always be treated promptly.

Causes of hypoglycaemia

Common causes of hypoglycaemia include:

- overadministration of insulin (p.19) or sulphonylurea tablets (p.26) (wrong dose prescribed or administered)
- excess of insulin (p.19) or sulphonylurea tablets (p.26) in relation to carbohydrates (p.9) (delayed or missed meals, reduced food intake)
- unplanned exercise (p.16)/increased physical activity (p.50)
- excess alcohol (p.14)
- heat (erratic blood glucose (p.42))
- cessation of steroid therapy (causes of hyperglycaemia (p.34))
- weight (p.17) loss
- hepatic/renal failure
- breastfeeding.

It is essential to identify/remedy the cause(s) of hypoglycaemia, making medication (p.19) adjustments where necessary, and providing appropriate education and self-management (p.8) support with a view to prevention (p.41). The diabetes team can assist with this.

Symptoms

When blood glucose levels fall to around 3.2 mmol/L, central nervous system-mediated symptoms are triggered which provide people with early warning signs. If blood glucose levels continue to fall below 3 mmol/L, the brain becomes starved of glucose, triggering additional symptoms which can be dangerously confused with drunkenness.

EARLY WARNINGS	FOLLOWED BY
Sweating, tingling, trembling, hunger, palpitations, pallor, anxiety, tachycardia	Blurred vision, difficulty speaking, confusion, dizziness, drowsiness, irritability, bizarre behaviour, fatigue, irrational agitation, paraesthesia, combativeness, coma

Experience of hypoglycaemic symptoms may be very individual. Some people with persistent <u>hyperglycaemia</u> (p.33) experience symptoms when their blood glucose levels fall, even though they may still be in the normal range. Gradually reducing their blood glucose levels over time will help them readjust to symptoms at more normal levels.

Hypoglycaemic unawareness

Long-standing diabetes and recurrent hypoglycaemic episodes can contribute to a loss of early warning signs, known as <u>hypoglycaemic unawareness</u>. This is dangerous because the features of more advanced hypoglycaemia can prevent people from making an appropriate response. Hypoglycaemic awareness can sometimes be restored if further hypos are prevented.

Nocturnal hypoglycaemia

Sometimes people with diabetes can have undetected hypos overnight. Indicators include raised fasting blood glucose levels ('rebound' <u>hyperglycaemia</u> (p.33)), night sweats, vivid dreams/nightmares and feeling groggy on waking. Testing blood glucose levels at 0300 hours can help rule these out.

People on intermediate/mixed <u>insulin</u> (p.19) may need a bedtime snack (plain biscuits, toast, cereal) to prevent nocturnal hypoglycaemia.

Treatment

Any blood glucose reading <4 mmol/L should be treated as a 'hypo'. Treatment will depend on severity but the principles are to use quick-acting <u>carbohydrates</u> (p.9) to raise the level above 4 mmol/L, before following on with long-acting carbohydrates (plain biscuits, toast, cereal, sandwich and planned meal) to prevent a further fall.

Inappropriate treatment, e.g. milk and a biscuit or a Mars® bar, is still prevalent and should be discouraged. Anything other than quick-acting carbohydrate, such as <u>fat</u> (p.12) and <u>fibre</u> (p.12), slows down the initial release of glucose, thereby delaying the return of normal blood glucose.

Mild to moderate hypos

Where people are still fully conscious, able to swallow and cooperate with treatment, administer 15–20g of quick-acting carbohydrate, e.g. approximately:

- 4–6 dextrose tablets
- 90–115 ml Lucozade®
- 150–200 ml cola or other full sugar fizzy drink
- 150–200 ml orange juice
- 3–4 jelly babies
- 3–4 wine gums
- 3–4 teaspoons of sugar
- 4–6 teaspoons of jam
- 20–30 ml Polycal.

Test blood glucose levels after 10–15 minutes and continue administering quick-acting carbohydrate until they are

≥4 mmol/L before administering long-acting carbohydrate. If this is not possible within three attempts, involve the medical team.

More severe hypos

Where people are still conscious but unable to swallow safely, 15–20g of quick-acting carbohydrate in the form of dextrose gel may be rubbed into the gums. When people are unconscious, treatment is either once-only intramuscular injection of 1mg glucagon (which releases glycogen stores from the liver/muscles – it can take up to 15 minutes to work and vomiting may occur) or intravenous dextrose according to local policy. Severe hypos may be accompanied by fitting or aggression. Always protect the airway.

Follow-on

Do not routinely withhold insulin (p.19)/other therapies (p.26) after a hypo – once treatment has restored normal blood glucose, diabetes medication may be administered when it is next due. It is, however, always important to address the causes of hypoglycaemia (p.38) and adjust medication appropriately if necessary.

Prevention

Every effort should be made to prevent hypoglycaemia. Not only is it unpleasant and frightening, it is also associated with poor clinical outcomes and cognitive impairment. Fear of hypoglycaemia encourages some people to prefer hyperglycaemia (p.33), thereby increasing their risk of long-term complications (p.44). Seek advice promptly from the specialist team for unexplained, prolonged or recurrent hypoglycaemia.

■ ERRATIC BLOOD GLUCOSE

A number of factors can contribute to erratic glycaemic control, including:

- variable carbohydrates (p.9)/meal timings
- inconsistent timing/dose(s) of diabetes medication (p.19)
- fluctuating exercise (p.16) levels
- poor injection technique
- lipohypertrophy (injection sites (p.25))
- temperature – heat (hot weather, bath, sauna) can speed up the absorption of insulin; excessive cold may slow it down.

The consequences of erratic blood glucose levels can be more severe in older people (p.49) and in children and young people (p.47), as well as in people who live on their own or have learning disabilities/mental health problems. It is important to identify and manage the cause(s) appropriately, making medication (p.19) adjustments as required, and providing education and self-management (p.8) support. If necessary, refer to the specialist team.

■ INPATIENT CARE

For people with diabetes, hospitalisation can have a significant impact on their diabetes – and vice versa – whether their admission is diabetes-related or not. Poor glycaemic control may prevent elective surgery/procedures or adversely affect outcomes, while factors that can affect blood glucose levels in hospital include:

- perioperative fasting
- disrupted medication (p.19)
- reduced appetite/change of diet (p.9)

- vomiting/diarrhoea
- change of exercise (p.16) level
- (par)enteral feeding
- infection
- surgery
- steroids.

Optimising glycaemic control during an inpatient stay can aid recovery and reduce morbidity. More frequent monitoring (p.30) may be required, as may adjustments to diabetes medication (p.19). Be alert to:

- persistent hyperglycaemia (p.33) with blood glucose levels >11 mmol/L
- recurrent and unexplained hypoglycaemia (p.38), especially with hypoglycaemic unawareness (p.39)
- erratic blood glucose (p.42) levels.

Always ensure people with diabetes in hospital are offered suitable meals/snacks at appropriate times and that their medication (p.19), if not self-administered, is given safely, at the correct dose and at the correct time.

Extended periods of fasting may require cover with a variable rate intravenous insulin infusion (VRIII). Different VRIII protocols exist – ensure the relevant protocol is followed exactly to avoid damaging blood glucose excursions. Protocols should also be followed for the management of myocardial infarction (MI), which carries special considerations.

Where problems arise, do not delay in contacting the diabetes team – timely referrals can significantly improve outcomes and help prevent discharge delays.

Long-term complications

Over time, diabetes is associated with the development of micro- and macrovascular changes in the body, which can lead to a number of serious irreversible pathologies, reducing life expectancy and quality of life for people with diabetes. The prevention (p.45) and care of these long-term complications is an important extension of diabetes management (p.7).

Figure 5 How diabetes complications affect the body

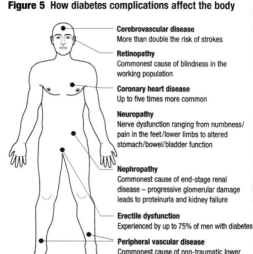

Cerebrovascular disease
More than double the risk of strokes

Retinopathy
Commonest cause of blindness in the working population

Coronary heart disease
Up to five times more common

Neuropathy
Nerve dysfunction ranging from numbness/pain in the feet/lower limbs to altered stomach/bowel/bladder function

Nephropathy
Commonest cause of end-stage renal disease – progressive glomerular damage leads to proteinuria and kidney failure

Erectile dysfunction
Experienced by up to 75% of men with diabetes

Peripheral vascular disease
Commonest cause of non-traumatic lower limb amputations

■ PREVENTION

The risk of developing long-term diabetes complications may be reduced, and their progression delayed, by:

- good <u>glycaemic control</u> (p.30)
- a healthy <u>lifestyle</u> (p.8)
- active management of cardiovascular risk factors, particularly blood pressure and blood lipids
- regular <u>screening and monitoring</u> (p.45)
- good <u>footcare</u> (p.46).

■ SCREENING AND MONITORING

Everyone with diabetes should be screened regularly for the development/deterioration of long-term complications as part of their <u>annual review</u> (p.29), with prompt follow-up treatment/onward referral and <u>self-management</u> (p.8) support as required.

Routine screening should cover:

- eye examination for retinopathy using digital retinal photography
- foot assessment for neuropathy and peripheral vascular disease
- blood and urine tests for nephropathy (glomerular filtration rate, serum creatinine, albumin:creatinine ratio)
- assessment of erectile dysfunction.

Routine monitoring should cover:

- <u>HbA_{1c}</u> (p.30) (6-monthly) for assessment of long-term glycaemic control
- blood pressure (6-monthly) – ideally aiming for <130/80 mmHg with angiotensin-converting enzyme (ACE) inhibitors/angiotensin II receptor blockers (ARBs) the antihypertensives of choice for their known protection

against coronary heart disease, nephropathy and retinopathy

- blood lipids – aiming for total cholesterol <4 mmol/L and triglyceride <1.7 mmol/L – with statin/antithrombotic therapy as required to protect against cardiovascular disease.

For children with diabetes, most screening/monitoring measures apply from age 12, with regular HbA$_{1c}$ from diagnosis.

Where problems arise, reviews may need to be more frequent. Be alert to the presence of diabetes complications and ensure any new or poorly managed symptoms/risk factors are followed up promptly.

■ FOOTCARE

A seemingly trivial problem can rapidly escalate to the point of emergency in the presence of ischaemic/neuropathic deficits in the diabetic foot/lower limb. The importance of footcare cannot be overemphasised.

- Wash feet daily and dry well, checking thoroughly for signs of damage or infection
- Keep nails short, carefully cutting or filing straight across to prevent damage and the risk of ingrowing nails
- Moisturise feet to keep skin supple and healthy
- Take care with baths, hot water bottles, etc. – reduced sensitivity may mask excessive heat
- Wear comfortable well-fitting footwear at all times, even indoors, to protect feet and prevent injury

Report any signs of circulatory compromise/infection/loss of skin integrity without delay. Any wounds which do not heal should also be followed up.

Life with diabetes

Few aspects of day-to-day life are unaffected by diabetes and the challenge of living with it extends to family and friends.

■ CHILDREN AND YOUNG PEOPLE

Although dedicated multidisciplinary paediatric teams provide intensive specialist input from the outset, a diagnosis of type 1 diabetes (p.3) in children or young people can be devastating for the whole family, requiring major adjustment and the rapid acquisition of self-management (p.8) skills.

With good familial support, many children adapt remarkably well but adolescence can be a difficult time with hormonal changes/emotional development impacting on glycaemic control. Young people finding their feet and asserting their independence may not always look after themselves very well and they may 'rebel' against their diabetes to their detriment (long-term complications (p.44)). Some omit insulin (p.19) to prevent weight gain, putting themselves at risk of diabetic ketoacidosis (DKA) (p.35), and eating disorders can be more common into adulthood. Psychological support may be required.

Not all young people attend their clinic appointments regularly and may face repeated hospital admissions. Be alert to the needs of this age group and aim to provide input and support to both the individuals and their families where opportunities present.

■ CULTURAL BACKGROUND

Different cultural groups have different perceptions and beliefs about life, about health and about diabetes. Religious rituals and festivals are a feature of every culture and some, e.g. fasting during Ramadan, may seem difficult to reconcile with recommended diabetes management (p.7). Be alert to potential cultural barriers and aim to address them with appropriate support, drawing on specialist input as required.

■ DEPRESSION

People with diabetes may be two to three times more likely to experience depression than the general population and this can have an adverse effect on glycaemic control (p.30) with reduced activity, comfort eating and alcohol consumption (lifestyle (p.8)). Be alert to signs of depression and provide advice/support as appropriate.

■ DRIVING

Most people with diabetes can continue to drive providing there are no debarring problems with hypoglycaemia (p.38) or long-term complications (p.44). Even people on insulin (p.19) may now apply for a licence to drive group 2 vehicles (lorries and buses) if they satisfy the criteria.

Insurance companies should be notified at diagnosis (this should not affect the premium), but the Driver and Vehicle Licensing Agency does not require notification unless diabetes medication (p.19) has been prescribed or health issues apply.

Drivers on insulin (p.19)/sulphonylurea tablets (p.26) should carry hypo treatment in the car at all times and conscientious monitoring (p.30) around journeys is essential to prevent hypoglycaemia (p.38) at the wheel.

■ EMPLOYMENT

It is illegal for employers to discriminate against people with diabetes in the workplace. Informing immediate colleagues and providing them with some basic education is a good idea so they can help in an emergency (hyperglycaemia (p.33), hypoglycaemia (p.38)).

■ END OF LIFE

For people receiving palliative care, diabetes management (p.7) is aimed at patient comfort/quality of life. This may result in a reduction, or even withdrawal, of medication (p.19) and monitoring (p.30). Advice from the specialist team may be helpful.

■ IDENTIFICATION

In case of emergency, people with diabetes should carry a diabetes identification card at all times, especially if they are on insulin (p.19).

■ NON-CONCORDANCE

Not everyone with diabetes succeeds in engaging with it positively and taking ownership. Many people do not follow lifestyle (p.8) advice and many do not take their prescribed medication (p.19). Be alert to the role of non-concordance in poor glycaemic control (p.30) and provide education/self-management (p.8) support where opportunities present.

■ OLDER PEOPLE

The prevalence of diabetes increases with age and diabetes management (p.7) in older people with complex co-morbidities/medication regimens is not always easy. Be alert to the risk of undetected hypoglycaemia (p.38) in older people living alone or in residential care. Also be alert to symptoms of diabetes (p.4) in anyone not known to have the condition.

Take every opportunity to reinforce diabetes education among staff in care settings.

■ PHYSICAL ACTIVITY

Exercise (p.16) is routinely encouraged as part of a healthy lifestyle but, for people on insulin (p.19), maintaining safe blood glucose levels around physical activity can be a challenge, involving frequent capillary blood glucose (CBG) (p.31) testing and adjustment of insulin doses/carbohydrates (p.9).

Exercise should never be attempted if blood glucose levels are:

- ≥14 mmol/L with ketones (p.33) – if there is not enough circulating insulin, stress hormones released by exercise may precipitate diabetic ketoacidosis (DKA) (p.35)
- <4 mmol/L without taking carbohydrates first (hypoglycaemia) (p.38).

Different types of exercise have different effects and individuals vary in their response to exercise. The specialist team can provide guidance. Advise people to carry hypo treatment and diabetes identification (p.49) at all times.

■ PREGNANCY

Pregnancy in women with diabetes carries a number of serious risks for mother and baby, including miscarriage, birth trauma, stillbirth and neonatal death. For women with pre-existing diabetes, the key to a healthy pregnancy is preconceptual planning with early optimisation of glycaemic control (HbA$_{1c}$ (p.30) <43 mmol/mol [6.1%]). For both pre-existing and gestational diabetes (types of diabetes (p.2)), tight glycaemic control throughout pregnancy is essential under joint obstetric/diabetes specialist care (NICE 2008).

■ PRESCRIPTIONS

Anyone with diabetes who has been prescribed diabetes <u>medication</u> (p.19) is entitled to free prescriptions.

■ SPECIAL OCCASIONS

People with diabetes do not have to forego special occasions. One-off rises in blood glucose levels from a celebratory night out will not affect their risk of developing <u>long-term complications</u> (p.44), but it is important not to let 'treats' become the norm. For eating out, recommend healthier <u>diet</u> (p.9) choices, portion control and moderate <u>alcohol</u> (p.14).

■ SUPPORT

Diabetes UK, the national charity which promotes diabetes care in the UK, is an excellent source of practical support for <u>self-management</u> (p.8). As well as publishing a range of literature in a variety of languages, Diabetes UK has an excellent website with a dedicated section for healthcare professionals. It runs a telephone helpline and also provides an advocacy service. Membership provides access to regular publications and updates about the condition.

■ TRAVEL

A good travel insurance policy that covers diabetes is essential. After that, the key is being well prepared. Advise people to take extra <u>monitoring</u> (p.30) and <u>medication</u> (p.19) supplies, as much as double anticipated needs, to avoid problems in the event of delays or lost luggage.

For air travel, <u>insulin</u> (p.19)/<u>glucagon-like peptide-1 (GLP-1) analogues</u> (p.28) should be carried in the cabin, not in the hold where they can freeze and become unusable (purpose-designed cool wallets are available to keep them at the correct temperature). The GP or diabetes team will provide documentation for airport security.

For long-haul journeys, the timing of medication is not always as complicated as it sounds. Always advise people to carry enough <u>carbohydrates</u> (p.9) to cover every eventuality – transport delays are common, mealtimes can be erratic and portion sizes may vary. Hot weather can contribute to <u>erratic blood glucose</u> (p.42) levels and more frequent <u>monitoring</u> (p.30) may be required. If people fall ill while away, they should follow <u>sick-day rules</u> (p.37).

■ VACCINATIONS

Any illness can have an adverse effect on <u>glycaemic control</u> (p.30) in people with diabetes. Pneumococcal and annual influenza vaccinations are recommended, along with appropriate <u>travel</u> (p.51) immunisations.

Glossary

----

acidosis   disturbance in the body's normal acid–base balance with increased acidity (<u>diabetic ketoacidosis [DKA]</u> (p.35))

basal–bolus regimen	combination of background (basal) and mealtime (bolus) insulin (p.19) in multiple daily injections (<u>blood glucose regulation (p.1)</u>)
glucagon	hormone produced by the pancreas that stimulates the release of stored glycogen from the liver/muscles when blood glucose is low (<u>blood glucose regulation (p.1)</u>)
glucometer	short for glucose meter, device for <u>capillary blood glucose (CBG) (p.31)</u> testing
<u>glycaemic control (p.30)</u>	blood glucose control
glycaemic index	scale ranking <u>carbohydrates (p.9)</u> according to their effect on blood glucose levels
glycogen	storage form of glucose in humans (<u>blood glucose regulation (p.1)</u>)
glycosuria	presence of glucose in the urine (<u>urinalysis (p.33)</u>)
<u>HbA$_{1c}$ (p.30)</u>	venous blood test used as a measure, in mmol/mol, of long-term <u>glycaemic control (p.30)</u>; previously quoted as a percentage
<u>hyperglycaemia (p.33)</u>	high blood glucose level, especially >11 mmol/L (<u>diagnosis (p.6)</u>)
hyperosmolarity	abnormally increased solute (osmolar) concentration (<u>hyperosmolar hyperglycaemic state [HHS] (p.36)</u>)

<u>hypoglycaemia</u> (p.38)	low blood glucose level
<u>insulin</u> (p.19)	hormone produced by the pancreas that enables body tissues to take up glucose from the bloodstream for use or storage as energy (<u>blood glucose regulation</u> (p.1))
insulin resistance	reduced sensitivity to the action of insulin associated in particular with central obesity and <u>lifestyle</u> (p.8) issues
ketonuria	presence of <u>ketones</u> (p.33) in the urine
lipohypertrophy	development of fatty lumps in subcutaneous tissue through overuse of <u>injection sites</u> (p.25)/reuse of needles
osmotic diuresis	increased urine output caused by the presence of glucose in fluid filtered by the kidneys (<u>symptoms of diabetes</u> (p.4))
polydipsia	excessive thirst leading to increased fluid intake (<u>symptoms of diabetes</u> (p.4))
polyuria	increased frequency and volume of micturition (<u>symptoms of diabetes</u> (p.4))
renal threshold	blood glucose level above which osmotic diuresis will occur, usually around 10 mmol/L

References

British National Formulary, www.bnf.org.uk.

NICE (2008) *Diabetes in pregnancy*, CG63, London: NICE.

Upton, D. (2010) *Student nurse health promotion survival guide*, Harlow: Pearson Education Ltd.

WHO (2006) *Definition and diagnosis of diabetes mellitus and intermediate hyperglycaemia*, Geneva: WHO.

WHO (2011) *Use of glycated haemoglobin (HbA$_{1c}$) in the diagnosis of diabetes mellitus*, Geneva: WHO.

Key documents

NICE (2011) *Diabetes in adults quality standard*, London: NICE.

NICE (2009) *Type 2 diabetes*, CG87, London: NICE.

NICE (2006) *Obesity*, CG43, London: NICE.

NICE (2004) *Type 1 diabetes*, CG15, London: NICE.

Department of Health (2001) *National service framework for diabetes*, London: Department of Health.

Useful websites

American Diabetes Association
www.diabetes.org

Diabetes UK
www.diabetes.org.uk

International Diabetes Federation
www.idf.org

Juvenile Diabetes Research Foundation
www.jdrf.org.uk

NHS Diabetes
www.diabetes.nhs.uk

Shift roster

DAY	DATE	SHIFT
MONDAY		
TUESDAY		
WEDNESDAY		
THURSDAY		
FRIDAY		
SATURDAY		
SUNDAY		